Supercharged Fitness For Seniors

Mirsad Hasic

DEDICATION

I dedicate this book to my wife.

CONTENTS

ACKNOWLEDGMENTS

I would like to thank my family for their support.

Introduction

January is truly an interesting month. Indeed, it is the only month that faces the past and the present at the same time. To me, that represents the fork in the road that most seniors face when it's time to start talking about health.

Do you go back to what's familiar, or do you blaze a new trail? Facing health often means that we have to face other aspects of our lives that we're ignoring. For many seniors, this means that we have to think about ourselves for a while rather than thinking about everyone else.

This is a time where the children aren't children anymore, but capable adults that usually have their own children to look after.

The joy of grandchildren running through the house is nice, but what's even better is having better health. Imagine being able to run and play with your grandchildren, or keep up with a few hobbies. Who said that getting old meant that you stopped playing?

So many people have written to me over the last few years about how they would love to take up a new active hobby but they just aren't sure that their bodies are up to the task. Or if they're confident that they can get in better shape, they just need a program that lets them be creative...within the rules, of course.

I'm just the person for the job. For the last few years I've been writing books on how to tailor the world of health to your needs.

I think it's high time that people took charge of their health, their bodies, and their desires for the future. It's totally okay to want to protect your body now so that you really can make the next decade or two as golden as possible.

We do that by looking deeper into health, making sure that we have a roadmap for success, and being willing to take consistent action no matter how hard it gets.

If you're focused on the same things, then I happily invite you to join me. Read this book and build your own success plan. I've laid out a full template to help you do that.

From time to time, you'll feel alone...even if a group of supportive people. Go back to all of the wonderful reasons why you decided to seize control of your health, and the rest will fall into place.

To YOUR success,
Mirsad Hasic

On Eating Well

What does it mean to eat well? Do you imagine glittering buffets and a free for all type of experience? Believe me, I'm not judging in the slightest.

Before I got serious about my health and what it meant to me, I could clear a buffet tray with the best of them.

I found myself in college without a lot of direction in the nutrition department. I knew I played soccer, I knew I was busy, and I knew that I wanted to keep enjoying the social life I had managed to build.

College was about class, friends, and figuring out life. I wasn't sure where I was going just yet, but I knew I wanted to be around for a long time.

You see, people often discount how short life is when they're young. I can honestly say that when I was in college, I really didn't think about it.

Unfortunately, the loss of a few good friends showed me that life can get cut short in the blink of an eye.

It also encouraged me to get serious about not being lazy. Yes, I just said the "L" word. You see, we all have gotten some lecture at some point in our lives about not being lazy.

Procrastination costs us in more ways than one. I used to work with someone that always had a reason why they couldn't do something on time.

It got to the point that they couldn't really reach their goals when everything was turned in late. I had a lot of friends in college with this problem.

They ended up falling behind in their studies and couldn't stay at university anymore. There is a better way than procrastination: planning, and taking ownership of your goals fully.

In the case of your health, it means getting serious about what you want. If you're looking for weight loss, as most seniors are, then you have to go beyond the whole "salad and water" approach.

A lot of people tend to heavily restrict calories, turning food into a punishment and a distant reward all at the same time. If only you could just stick to the diet for a while, then you could treat yourself to all of those amazing dishes your family makes every year.

The truth is that if you're flexible, you can have the best of both worlds. It's like getting to ride the roller coaster and then moving over to the bumper cars at an amusement park...with just enough time left over to jump into the pool to cool down. (1)

Now, the twists and turns of losing weight involve our current mindset, plus how we respond and react to other people. The first roadblock to get over is that of constant approval.

The opinions of other people don't need to play a heavy role in your health. If you know that you would like to lose weight, then you need to put steps in place that allow you to achieve that goal.

In a nutshell, eating well is less about volume and more about purpose. So the guide below is about selection and getting the best quality that you can afford, without punishing yourself for what you can't have at the moment.

This is primarily a low carb framework, with Flex Days and Focus Days. The way it works is straightforward: on a flex day you can eat more foods that are higher in carbohydrates, but still as whole as possible.

A sweet potato with a bit of sour cream, leeks, meat, and cheese is a far better choice for your health plan than it would be to eat a ton of pizza and ice cream.

On a Focus Day, you need to do exactly what it says on the proverbial tin: focus on eating the foods that are going to help you power through your day. What are those foods, you might ask? I have you covered below.

Start with Fat

Starting with fat is wise because it helps round out your food framework. One of the toughest problems that people have with staying on a particular diet is that they tend to get hungry.

When they get hungry, they're going to go for the quickest thing they can eat in order to get rid of that hunger feeling. Usually finger foods that are easy to eat are also high in carbohydrates.

What is a savvy senior to do when they're trying to improve performance? Turn to increased fat intake, of course! Everything has pros and cons, so let's go with the pros and cons of increasing this necessary nutrient.

Pros

Fat helps in the production of hormones. Fat soluble vitamins require sufficient fat intake in order for those vitamins to be used within the body. Failure to get the right amounts can result in losing performance, rather than gaining it. So the bottom line is that fat really is a good thing for us. (2), (3)

Cons

If you have gallbladder problems, upping your fat intake might take more time than someone who has a functioning gallbladder.

You may need to talk with your doctor about what you need to do next.

However, I've found that many of my friends have benefited from adding digestive enzymes that help them break down fat. That way, they get the benefits of increasing their fat consumption without making digestion a painful thing. (4)

Great sources of fat include: butter, lard, chicken fat, turkey fat, coconut oil, olive oil, and tallow. Coconut oil is really good because it has MCTs (medium chain triglycerides) that help the body metabolize nutrients for energy. (5)

You need to understand that fat is not a bad thing. The first thing that most senior citizens worry about when it comes to increasing fat intake would have to be saturated fat. They've been taught almost their entire lives that this is the "bad fat" that causes heart disease.

It's only recently that we've really begun to look at fat differently, even though the debate is decades old. The science currently points to saturated fat being more protective rather than destructive.

Hormone production is the key to our health, and there are way too many hormone reactions that depend on adequate fat intake. So the low fat diet faze is actually more dangerous than increasing fat intake. What are you leaving on the table due to bad health advice? (6), (7)

Cholesterol is so important to the body that we produce it naturally, partially from what we eat but more from internal processes.

You don't want to skip adding in cholesterol from saturated fat, because it's only going to aid in your body's overall performance. (8)

Trouble in Paradise

At this point, you might wonder why I didn't mention certain oils. You should know ahead of time that not everything is good for you, even if it's found in the supermarket.

Remember that this world is set up often on bad advice, which means that people are making money off bad health without really realizing it. But that's a topic for a far different book.

I'm more concerned with your health, so I will explain why some oils are beneficial and others are destructive. Take canola oil, for example. It's readily available in just about every grocery store, but is it really good for us? Not at all. (9), (10)

The reason why is simple: it oxidizes easily. Open your fridge right now and smell some of your leftovers. That off smell that you get from food barely a day old isn't the food itself, but the oil that it's cooked in.

Canola oil is a heavily refined oil that is high in omega 6 fatty acids, an essential fatty acid that the body needs but not at the same levels that it needs omega 3 fatty acids.

Taking in oxidized oils actually encourages the production of free radicals that end up aging our bodies from the inside out.

All of the antioxidants in the world aren't helpful if we keep taking in substances that cause more free radicals. We need to heal our bodies by eating fewer oils that are high in omega 6 and switch to foods that have more omega 3.

You'll find rich sources of omega 3 when you turn to grass-fed beef and wild caught seafood, but the conventional versions of these foods still pack a nice punch.

You can also supplement as well with fermented cod liver oil, but this isn't an absolute necessary if you're getting rid of the excess omega 6. The body will eventually correct over time. (11)

Protein Options

I love meat, eggs, seafood...you name it, and I enjoy it! There's just something about coming from work and looking in my slow cooker at the roast that's been slowly getting tender while I've been gone. I'm a huge believer in better health, but I don't have time to be chained to the stove.

I need to be able to get my priority tasks done and be able to still eat well. It's possible that you already have a slow cooker available, but if you don't they are very affordable. I can't quote you specific prices, but I've found a lot of budget friendly options out there.

If you're in a hurry, I always recommend eggs for their affordability as well as their versatility. You can add eggs to just about anything and still get a tasty meal.

They're even delicious on their own with just a little bit of cream and spices. (12)

As an aside, I encourage you to find herbs and spices that pair well with things that fit on your framework. Whether it's a flex day or a focus day, you should feel empowered to make your food taste good. After all, if you don't find it appealing, you won't eat it. That would ruin the point of a food framework, right?

Pros

Protein is very satisfying, especially when it's paired with fats. If you load up on protein, you'll find that it doesn't take nearly as much protein to feel full. Compare that to the average serving of carbohydrates, and how we feel after the meal.

Usually after a meal that's heavy on the carbohydrates, there's a temporary feeling of satisfaction. But as the blood sugar roller coaster winds up again, that feeling of happiness is very short lived. (13)

Cons

Some people don't like a lot of meat in their diets, or have been told to cut down on it. Even if you don't like things like pork, you could always switch to turkey. If you don't want to deal with land animals at all, why not take a look at seafood?

Another downside of increasing your protein intake is that there is a bit of a cost difference between most carbohydrates and most proteins. It's not hard to see that proteins are often the most expensive category in the supermarket today, but there are ways to get things cheaper. You can be on the lookout for discounts and coupons, along with sharing the costs with friends. This would involve having a local farm that you can buy meat from, but there could be one hiding very close to home. (14)

Delicious Veggies

This plan doesn't work without vegetables, in my opinion. You need to get in a good amount of fiber in order to maintain good digestion, and veggies add a certain layer of flavor to just about every dish.

If you don't like most vegetables cooked, you might prefer them raw. I have a few friends that I wouldn't dare serve cooked vegetables to because they really like the feel of the raw version.

Great veggies abound for the low carb framework: cabbage, cauliflower, broccoli, carrots, onions, peppers, salad greens of all stripes, and plenty more. There are free lists of carb counts for vegetables, and it would be wise to jot down a few figures. The reason why I'm not listing all of them for you is simple:

I want you to get in the habit of looking up this information. If you're going to track your food regularly, then you need to get used to looking up nutritional values.

People that are coming into this from a low fat framework might be a bit shocked by the fact that they need to track carb intake rather than fat grams, but the transition is a lot smoother than you think. It's much easier to track carbs rather than fat, and much healthier in the long run! (15)

Pros

Veggies are a great source of fiber, and it helps maintain regular digestive patterns. If you're worried about constipation, regular veggie consumption will help combat this embarrassing and painful condition. Vegetables also cut down on free radicals by giving the body valuable antioxidants like Vitamin C.

Magnesium and potassium are also found in many vegetables. These two nutrients are key factors in helping the body maintain the necessary balance for vibrant living. If you're worried about blood pressure, magnesium is extremely important.

Cons

If you were a picky eater in the past, it might be hard to increase your veggie intake. But there are really so many different ways to prepare vegetables that you owe it to yourself to give it another try.

You can fry, steam, bake, roast and even combine veggies with other ingredients to make a really awesome casserole. The carbohydrates you'll find in veggies are mostly fiber, making them an ideal choice for low carb frameworks like this one.

Dairy Dreams

Dairy is a hot-button issue for some. Many low carb framework fans enjoy dairy. When it's full fat rather than the low fat variety, it's a filling and nutritious part of a food plan.

Unfortunately, not everyone can afford to add dairy to their diet. Some people are extremely adverse to dairy and have bad stomach problems from it. I'm one of those people that can enjoy some dairy, but not a lot before I experience problems.

So I try to use dairy products as an accent in my cooking rather than a heavy part of it. There are dairy-free options that use coconut milk, which would also double as a fat source. (16)

Dairy sources include milk, cottage cheese, ricotta cheese, hard cheeses like cheddar and Swiss, yogurt, ice cream (sugar-free varieties sweetened with Splenda are a nice treat) and sour cream. Most grocery stores have affordable varieties, so it's never a bad idea to investigate what works for you.

This is the reason why I suggest tracking your food: if you do have food intolerances, you can see exactly where they are and remove those foods right away. If you're just eating mindlessly without really thinking about it, then you run into problems with figuring out what might be the problem. (17)

Pros

Dairy is incredible flavorful, with a creamy texture that we can't wait to enjoy. It's nice to enjoy as part of a great framework, if you can handle it. I like to mix sour cream into eggs while scrambling them for a really fluffy end-product. And when I mention eggs, you should remember to use the whole egg with that golden yolk in the mix! :)

Cons

The biggest downside to dairy is that some people absolutely cannot tolerate it. That doesn't mean that they have to get rid of the rest of the framework, but that they can't have dairy involved.

It's easy to avoid dairy as long as you're reading labels, which you should do anyway. Knowing what's going into your food is a good idea and will help you stay on plan. Don't be afraid to ask in restaurants what everything is made of as well. (18)

What to Avoid

If we're going to talk about the things that you can have, we have to talk about the things that you need to avoid. Now, I don't think that you have to avoid all of these foods forever.

For example, I generally steer people away from whole oats because of the high carb amount. However, you may want to include this on your Flex days. If you handle oats well, this might be something you look into. However, it's very easy to go beyond your desired carb limits very quickly with these foods. (19)

One of the first foods I tell people to avoid would have to be things made from flour. It's high carbs without much nutrition at all. Most of the nutrients in refined white flour are from the fortification process rather than being naturally wholesome.

Excessive carb intake causes a sharp blood sugar response, which is the last thing that we want. If you've already been diagnosed with diabetes, then you want to pay special attention to lowering your carb intake as much as possible.

Your doctor will be able to watch your improvements much better since they're working with you one on one. Let them know that you're using this framework as a way to control your blood sugar and avoid the wild fluctuations that make diabetes so difficult to deal with. (20), (21)

Another area of contention would have to be potatoes. White and sweet potatoes tend to get a bad rap, but they are perfect for your flex days. I say this because I know that there's often a lot of temptation to eat much more damaging foods.

If you have the choice between two medium sweet potatoes and an all-out fast food binge, I'm going to tell you to take the sweet potatoes and treat yourself, and then get back to the plan.

Remember that flex days aren't absolutely necessary; they're designed to serve you, not the other way around. This means that if you aren't served by flex days, you don't have to use them. But if you find that you need just a little bit of wiggle room, so to speak, you can try them out to see if it works for you. (22)

Tracking Tips

If you're going to take this bold step towards better health and increased physical performance, then we have to make consistent changes and be able to track those changes over time.

Tracking is essentially the "missing ingredient" that keeps so many people from their goals. The reason why might not be obvious, however.

You see, if you get into a nice routine but hit a roadblock in terms of weight loss, you don't know what to change. Without tracking, you can't go back and recall everything that you ate on a certain date.

A lot of people believe that they can remember things for long periods of time, but you might be shocked to find out just how short your memory really is!

In other words, if you plan for maximum success you need to track all of your food. It can get a little tricky if you eat out, because you have to try to find nutritional breakdowns of common dishes served at restaurants.

But if you apply more of a low carb approach to eating out, where you avoid things high in carbohydrates, you may find that you eat much more simply anyway.

You don't have to spend a lot of money on expensive software to track your food intake over the next few months.

A simple pen and paper will help you more than any software will. The habit formed by tracking things helps us focus, think about our goals, and be willing to make changes along the way. (23)

Modifying Your Food Plan

Changes are part of every single framework I can think of. Even on the famous Atkins program, moving to the last phases of the program means adding back in whole grains, but in a smaller concentration.

You're always looking at where your ideal carb intake level should be, rather than being in a static program.

The only way to really make sure that things are moving along is to have an accurate record, to the best of your ability, of what you're taking in.

Tracking works because it forces us to think mindfully about what we're eating. A lot of people, even senior citizens, tend to be so busy with moving from one problem to the next that they really don't stop and focus on anything in particular. Eating goes out the window, and we just fixate on what's going to be the fastest.

It's beyond time to slow down and think more about how we feel, what we eat, and if we really do enjoy what we're consuming.

Now, if you've read anything I've written in the past, you know that I feel like our culture encourages too much rushing around.

Don't get me wrong: I have a high work ethic, and I'm not afraid to push forward when I need to get things done.

But I never equate what I do with who I am, in the sense that my whole life will fall apart if I take a rest day. I have taken numerous life-changing trips, and plan to travel more in the future.

You've earned a chance to step back and evaluate any and all health frameworks that you're interested in. For the sake of this guide, I'll be giving you suggestions along the way that can help you refine this plan and make it more unique to your situation.

After all, it's not like I'm able to be right there next to you, even though I wish I could do that for all of my readers. Instead, I'm going to give you as much commentary, good sense, and facts that I can in order to get you back on track.

We all get derailed at one point or another, but that's all in the past. You're on a new path to success, and I'm committed to helping you get there...and stay there!

So, to recap this chapter:

- Eating well is the intersection of good food and good performance. When we have both pieces of the equation balanced, good health is surely around the corner.

- Do not feel like you have to start right away. It's perfectly fine to read through this framework, and make slow but consistent changes over a few weeks.

- If you have an allergy to any food, please do not consume it. Food intolerances and allergies play havoc with our immune response system, and the foods that don't play well with our systems should be avoided as much as possible. For example, if you are lactose intolerant, don't wander too far into dairy. Unsweetened coconut milk can be just as satisfying as the cow's milk that you are more accustomed to.

- Tracking your food doesn't have to be difficult. To make it easier, pick a time every day that you'll sit down for at least 15 minutes to jot it all down. If you have a smartphone, you can always leave an audio memo to yourself to listen to later.

Addressing Bone Health

It's time that we all started giving our bodies a break now and then, right? And I don't mean the type of break you get when you fall down the stairs. All puns aside, it's time to get serious about bone health.

After all, our bones don't really ask for much, and yet they handle movement every day and every night without much input from us. For most of us, it's a matter of putting one foot down in front of the other, and not stopping until you get to your destination. But what can we really do to protect the bones of the human body? (24)

The answer starts in learning a few things about the human skeletal system. You might have heard that we have 206 bones in the body, which is a long way from the nearly 300 bones that we have at birth.

Cartilage converts to bone, and we get that solid system we enjoy fully from our 20s all the way through till death.

Just as we can have strong bones, we also can have weak ones as well. Osteoporosis and low bone density can team up to weaken bones to the point of fracture, making it hard to get anything done. (25)

Does that mean that we have to have weak bones or simply sit on the sidelines because of arthritis? Not at all.

As we get older, it's only natural to find that our bodies have changed quite a bit. The human skeleton doesn't just weaken overnight, but there is some bone density loss due to lower mineral levels.

Calcium is only part of the problem here; there are other minerals that play a healthy role in keeping bones strong for a long time. In fact, sticking only with calcium is where most of the problems we deal with come from.

The picture is much more complex than just saying calcium for strong bones. When we were all younger, we had higher levels of activity that actually strengthened our bones. Did you know that the bones are constantly breaking down and being rebuilt, over and over again?

Our bodies are designed to heal themselves, but poor living stunts the healing process. Thankfully, once we're armed with the right information, we can do a lot to reverse this process. (26), (27)

Boosting Bone Health

As you go through this section, keep in mind that you may already have the proper levels of each mineral in your system. That said, it never hurts to learn more about the vitamins and minerals that can aid in better bone health.

The changes you're looking for won't happen overnight, of course. Yet it's important that once you change things for the better, the road ahead must include consistency and focus.

You can't focus on better bone health and then skip the supplementation later when you feel better. This will be lifelong process, and a permanent change.

Magnesium

A lot of people ignore the role of magnesium in the body, but we can't afford to make that same mistake. There are actually over 300 different chemical reactions that our bodies depend upon every day for optimal health that require magnesium.

These hormonal decisions can literally make the difference between a great life where you can thrive, and one where you're struggling to handle the everyday concerns of life. Magnesium is abundant in the body, but that doesn't mean that it sticks around forever.

It can be leached from the body due to stress, poor eating habits, excessive alcohol consumption and lack of sleep.

All of these things can play a role in how much magnesium you have in your body. Don't forget that magnesium is eliminated through urine, which is why it's important to have regular intake. (28)

If you're avoiding dairy because of intolerance, then you may be concerned that you can't get the magnesium you need. There's no need for alarm; you can supplement with magnesium chloride.

People that have Type 2 diabetes are susceptible to magnesium deficiencies, and if you already have this condition it would be wise to consult with your doctor about your desire to supplement with magnesium. While these tips should still serve you well, it's always best to let a doctor give you their opinion as a medical professional.

Of course, there are other groups that can be susceptible to magnesium loss. If you have celiac disease, Crohn's disease, alcohol dependence, or have had a gastric bypass operation, you want to pay close attention to your magnesium levels.

If you start feeling very fatigued, it could be a sign that your magnesium levels get depleted far faster than other people. You could also have problems absorbing the magnesium that you take in.

As we get older, our kidneys actually excrete more magnesium than they did when we were younger. This is why you have to stay as vigilant as possible on the matter.

Worried our food framework from earlier won't allow you to get the most magnesium possible? Don't worry. Avocado, spinach, bony fish and carrots all have magnesium.

Vitamin A

This vitamin isn't just good for aiding in vision health; our bones need adequate amounts of Vitamin A. You might have heard of this vitamin as retinol or beta-carotene.

Vitamin A helps in cell division as well as in cell differentiation. Retinol is near perfect for the body in its natural state, with not much for the body to do in order to be able to use it. Beta-carotene, on the other hand, needs a lot more processing in order to make it viable. Both forms of this vitamin are stored in the liver.

Now, here's the good news for those of us transitioning to a low carb diet: you can get your fair share of Vitamin A through animal foods and plants instead of processed foods.

The biggest thing that the low carb framework I outlined earlier brings to the table is that you start getting away from processed foods very quickly, if you decide to be diligent about following the framework. (29), (30)

Like most things in the body, too little or too much Vitamin A can lead to serious problems. You have to be careful not to overdo Vitamin A through use of retinol skin creams.

While many senior citizens are a bit conscious of their looks in terms of wrinkles and age spots, it's critical that you avoid using too many skin creams with retinol in them.

Although these preparations are synthetic, it's been shown to have similarly negative impact on bone health as dietary sources.

So while liver is a great source, you don't have to have chicken liver every week.

Beta-carotene can be consumed at a higher amount without worry of vision or bone problems. I recommend sticking to food sources, since the absorption rate is slower, giving your body time to process things.

Vitamin D

Think that all you need to do is lie in the sun and Vitamin D will make itself? Actually...you're right! Well, most of the time, that is. You see, Vitamin D is a very important substance for the body, and it's generated by being in direct sunlight.

You need real sun, not tanning beds in order to get the full effect. The ultraviolet rays of the sun directly begin the process. Yet if you are dark skinned, the body's melanin works as a shield against the sun. This is good for avoiding sunburns, but not so good for getting the Vitamin D that you need.

So if you're someone that can't be in the sun, has dark skin or is just very removed from sunny weather, it's time to think about supplementing.

The Vitamin D Council estimates that the majority of adults today are deficient in Vitamin D and just don't know it.

They are opening themselves to health risks and this needs to be addressed the entire year, not just in summer.

Living in Sweden has taught me that one cannot just rely on the sun to always be there. I supplement Vitamin D3 in the winter, and I recommend that you do the same. (31), (32)

Why D3, though? Vitamin D3 is known as cholecalciferol, and it's the form of the vitamin best synthesized and absorbed by the body. It's the form that we make from the sun, so it makes sense that we would supplement that form as well.

Vitamin D works well with vitamins A and K2, two other vitamins that you'll want to take into consideration.

If you're eating fatty fish like catfish, mackerel, sardines, tuna and herring, you're going to get a good amount of D3.

Fortified processed foods aren't a good source of Vitamin D3; most mass-produced products use the cheaper form that's absorbed readily by plants, but you're not a head of broccoli or a bunch of bananas on a tree. In other words, this isn't going to adjust your blood levels very much.

Did you know that aside from bone health, Vitamin D3 plays a big role in your body's immune system? Without a healthy immune system, it can feel like every single illness plagues you all the time.

You catch more colds than most people and you constantly feel run down. Some even say that when their bodies run low on D3 they can't think clearly and they also find themselves becoming more depressed with time. None of those things sound very good, and it's better to supplement as soon as you can.

There are simple blood tests that you can order to see how deficient you are, but the Vitamin D Council does assume a high percentage of adults are deficient already, hence they push for supplementation without too much delay.

Vitamin K2

Out of all of the vitamins and minerals that I've talked about in this section, vitamin K2 is probably one of the ones we ignore the most. But it's very necessary in the body, handling everything from bone health to better brain functionality.

As we age, cognitive function tends to get weaker, so anything we can do to boost brain power and bone health at the same time is a good thing.

You can find this vitamin naturally through fermented veggies like sauerkraut, kimchi, and natto. Goose liver is also rich in K2. If you can tolerate dairy, grass-fed butter has high K2 value. Organ meats tend to carry high K2 levels, but not everyone's comfortable eating kidneys and hearts. (33)

There are a few things that are very important to know before you begin supplementation. K2 is not K1; they are two very separate vitamins. Remember our good buddy calcium? In order for calcium to fully benefit the body, K2 levels have to be optimal.

Without this vital vitamin in your system, the regulation of calcium gets disrupted big time. Low levels of K2 impact the bones as well as the heart. Optimal levels of K2 improve bone mineral density, essentially keeping osteoporosis at bay.

You need to take all of these boosters together, rather than just addressing them separately. If you don't take A but you get lots of K2, you're going to have problems.

Everything works together for the good of the whole system, so lacking one means that you're creating a vacuum that has to be filled in.

So, to recap this chapter:

- We need to get proper vitamins and minerals in the body to maintain bone health.
- Good food intake from our low carb framework will help ensure that we get the minerals we need without all of the processed food we don't.
- While fortified foods can seem like a shortcut to getting better health, the vitamins and minerals added are often synthetic and of poor quality on a mass-produced product. Getting supplements that are made from quality materials is the way to go, and there are budget friendly options at every level.
- Remember to be consistent if you choose to go the supplementation route for bone health.

Managing Food Traditions

We don't really think of the time around the family dinner table as a tradition, but it most certainly is. Just about everyone can recall a time when everything the world was throwing at them just melted away in the presence of good food and great people.

Do all of those memories have to go away just because we're transitioning to a low carb diet?

Not at all. In order to move forward, however, you're going to have to take a hard look at the things that you used to eat and realize that you aren't going to be able to eat them in the same way.

There may be some modifications you can make, but the emotional toll this takes may be a lot more than what you bargained for.

Indeed, just about every family has a recipe that's often high in sugar and processed ingredients.

My aunt makes these amazing cookies but they're loaded with sugar and tend to be with cheap, processed flours.

Of course, when I got them in the mail at university I didn't complain about those things. I devoured the cookies with relish and decided that I'd just pretend that the weight increase was just due to college stress.

Do you already have a gaggle of grandchildren? They're probably used to cookies and cakes aplenty, which means that there's a conversation that needs to be had with your children before everyone comes over to visit. Bringing over all of these foods is only going to make you want to step off of your path.

Does that mean that everything is lost? Of course not! Your family will always be there, even if they don't really understand what you're doing. Some may feel that you're taking away all of the fun, because sometimes change is really hard to deal with.

But if you follow the tips below there may be some things that you can do to ease the tension before it spirals out of hand.

First and foremost, you need to let them know that they are welcome to eat anything they like. Even though it seems irrational, people tend to feel like you're criticizing their life decisions.

Your adult children may feel that you're trying to tell them what they're doing with their own children is wrong, which never goes over very well.

By affirming that you're making better choices for yourself, you're making it clear that they are free to do whatever they would like. But don't be surprised if they join in on your decision to make better health choices!

Next, you may want to invest in a few low carb recipe books. Cookbooks are a great way to cut down on the trial and error part of cooking and baking because someone else has already done that and written about their adventure!

I like to turn to cookbooks when I'm lost for ideas and company is coming over. While my wife and I like simple meals, I find that company is often wowed by more elaborate dishes.

Finally, keep the junk out of the house. This is the step that a lot of people fail because they figure that if they have "just one", they'll be okay. Folks, a lot of people absolutely cannot have just one cookie or one slice of cake.

They like the sweetness factor so much that they'll happily go in and get seconds, thirds, fourths...until the cake or pie dish is completely empty.

Then they feel bad about it the next day and the day after that, creating a cycle of bad feelings that haunt them until they end up making the same sugary decision again and again.

That's not a great way to live because you end up blaming yourself for problems that you didn't create and things that you never meant to really do.

There are some quick meals and treats that I tend to go back to often:

- Lettuce-wrapped sandwiches with vinaigrette dressings
- Huge salads with dark, leafy greens as the base and boiled eggs and strips of meat on top

- Simple mousses made with stevia or Splenda as the sweetener (hey, a good mousse uses eggs and raw cacao, with the latter ingredient being expensive enough that you won't overdo it)
- Sugar free jellos and puddings
- Roasted veggies
- The "guts" from eggrolls and tacos (meaning no bread products at all, just the ingredients inside a bowl with fork at the ready to eat)

I like to keep it simple because too many ingredients take time in the kitchen that could be spent enjoying the meal with the people I care about.

At the end of the day, you'll make new traditions as you enter a new phase in your life.

If the only reason everyone is visiting you is to get the latest cake or pie, then that's a sign that they care more about the food than they do about your company. Stand up for what you're choosing to do; you'll come out all right in the end.

Redefining Mobility

What does it mean to move well? Does it mean that we can run a marathon, or take on a few sprints like Usain Bolt?

The truth is somewhere a bit different: within our own hobbies, interests, and lifestyles. We need to be able to move around our world in order to interact, food delivery services notwithstanding. You have a lot more to gain from being able to seek out things on your own versus being chained to your bed.

While that isn't something I'm intimately familiar with many of the amazing individuals I chatted with while writing this book mentioned experiencing that type of low mobility, or seeing it in a loved one.

It is the ultimate torture to be able to move well and experience what life has to offer, only to find that people you love can't do the same. So we're going to explore mobility in this section and see what we can do to improve it, and also claim more of it for ourselves.

Mobility is basically how we move, as well as how well we move. Have you ever started a new exercise program, but felt like your bones and joints were going to come out of their sockets?

Chances are good that you didn't have a high degree of mobility, so all of the moves just ended up making you feel stiffer and stiffer.

Now, think of mobility like a rubber band. We can stretch a new rubber band better than a dried out band that has been sitting at the bottom of our junk drawer pile for a while. (34)

But let's dig a little deeper. Surely there are ways to improve mobility that don't involve us jumping in headfirst, right? Believe it or not, you can improve mobility by getting gradually more active.

It just depends on how active you were to begin with. For me, increasing activity would require far tougher tasks than someone that's been on the couch for a really long time. Starting out small doesn't mean that you'll remain there.

Suppose that you're someone that already has a fairly active life. In this case, I'm referring to the senior citizen that goes out to run their own errands and can stand at the kitchen counter chopping onions without necessarily getting tired.

This is a person that can raise their activity by continuing to stand up and move. Why is standing so powerful? In a word, it's this: our ancestors had to be upright for long periods of time. There was work to do out in the fields, and it took a lot of time to go out looking for food.

If we couldn't handle standing up for long stretches of time, we would have died out a long time ago. It's only through technology that we're able to sit around all day without paying a heavy cost for it. We don't have to go out and hunt our food, just go down to the supermarket. (35)

Other standing activities include:
- Preparing and cooking food
- Gardening
- Trimming the tree branches outside
- Taking care of runaway brush and bushes
- Rearranging lawn or yard furniture (tables, chairs, small stands)
- Lifting and cleaning picture frames
- Light to moderate housecleaning
- Ironing clothes
- Sorting clothes bound for the washer
- Hanging up wet clothes to dry on the clothesline

Standing improves blood circulation and encourages your muscles to move in the controlled fashion we're looking for. Remember that muscle movement is based on the "use it or lose it" system. If you don't move around, it will become very difficult to keep going over time.

Stretching for Mobility

When you want to continue to improve mobility, stretching should be at the top of your list. If you can stretch regularly, you'll be able to keep your muscles and joints in good working condition. Think about stretching the same way that people prepare their cars for winter driving.

Do they tend to just jump in, turn on the car, and take off? If they want their car to last for more than just one or two winters, they know that they have to let the car warm up first.

That's going to set the tone for the smoothest ride possible. I'm not trying to call you a machine, but there's a parallel here that you should consider. If we can stretch every day, then it will set the tone for more exercise.

You don't have to pull out any fancy stretches. I like yoga, but if you're not a huge fan of turning yourself into a pretzel, you don't have to do it. :) I'm a firm believer in the benefits of yoga, but that's not what I'm talking about here.

Just stand up and reach for the sky like you're trying to touch the sun. Bending down low like you're trying to reach for something on the group can help as well. I use both of these stretches all of the time.

If you're working at a desk on a project for long periods of time, these stretches will get your blood moving back to other constricted areas of the body.

When we sit for a while, our legs don't always get the blood circulation they really need. As blood rushes back in, you might feel a little bit tingly for a few minutes, but that feeling will go away as you stretch and move around.

Walking for Health

Good mobility and walking go hand in hand. I've seen people change their entire lives just from walking. If you want to eventually take advantage of the exercise methods I'll describe later in this book, improving mobility through walking is a great idea.

Try this "block by block" method to get started. Think about how far you could walk in terms of blocks. If you're on the metric system, you can think of this in kilometers if you like.

For my American audience, you're mostly thinking in miles, and that's perfectly fine. If you normally walk about 5 blocks comfortably, then start there. Every week, you'll need to add two more blocks. (36)

So it might look like this:
- **Week 1**: 5 blocks
- **Week 2**: 7 blocks
- **Week 3**: 9 blocks
- **Week 4**: 11 blocks

After 4 weeks, you may want to go up by three blocks rather than just two. This way you're still feeling challenged.

Of course, some people might start at 10 blocks or 15 blocks, and that's really great. Hey, there's always room for the advanced in the class. I'm here to challenge you no matter where you're starting from.

Mobility Maintenance

Just as you have to stretch, you also need to make sure that you're resting as much as you can. I'm not just talking about taking it easy from time to time, but getting enough sleep.

We'll touch on sleep in the next few chapters, but we can't skip over resting. It's when we're asleep that the body does most of its recovery efforts, rebuilding the muscle that we tear up through vigorous activity.

It might sound like you don't want to "tear" your muscles up like this, but it's really a good thing. If we don't challenge the body, we'll get weaker over time and well...you're already experiencing that to some degree, right?

If you wake up feeling like you're just not as young as you used to be, it's really a mobility issue hiding as an age issue. There are plenty of active senior citizens that lead very vibrant lives. Following the friendly advice in this guide can help make sure that you join them eventually. (37)

I like to go for a run in the mornings, and every week I challenge myself to go just a little bit farther.

A six mile run is a bit light, but I challenge myself by trying to run it faster than I did the week before. So it's not just a matter of distance for me, but also speed.

You might get to a point where speed of movement is important as well, or you might feel that this isn't a real priority. Work on distance first, and then let speed improve over time.

Walking regularly is also connected to lower levels of depression. It makes sense when you get to watch the world just wrap itself around you on your foot travels. It gives you time to work through any issues that you have going on, without all of the interruptions of everyday life.

Senior mental health is something that doesn't get talked about nearly enough. I understand that the people that came before me have gone through things I can't even imagine, and they're proud that they lived to tell the tale.

But this perspective is often accompanied by a strong sense of pride, and that pride easily can lead to not being willing to confront other issues in the background. If you feel like you have to keep it all bottled up, walking will help you release your feelings in a way that still doesn't involve a lot of people in your life.

However, I will say that if you feel like you're sinking; seeking professional counseling is nothing to be ashamed of. There are just some things that simple walking can't take away, you know? Don't be afraid to take care of yourself first and foremost!

So, to recap this chapter:

- Make mobility a priority, with regular stretching and standing.
- The more you stand, the more you condition your body to take on activity.

- Walking is not only a great way to promote weight loss, but it can also lower feelings of depression.
- Serious depression that doesn't go away should be handled by a professional, and I can't stress this enough.
- Give yourself plenty of time to walk and move around if you're not used to a lot of activity. It gets easier over time!

Sleep Fixes

Nearly everyone isn't getting enough sleep in order to face the challenges of everyday living. But if you really work at it, you can improve sleep hygiene to the point where you're getting not just more sleep, but much more restful sleep.

This is a very important difference that a lot of people just skip over. You must make sure that you're getting every advantage out of sleeping, so you're mentally and physically prepared for the challenges of the day.

It's been shown that when we don't get enough sleep, our cognitive functions are greatly reduced. In short, it's harder to think and it's even harder to motivate yourself to move around. In this section we'll work on what needs to be done in order to get the best sleep possible.

There's a common myth that seniors don't need as much sleep across the board, and that's not necessarily the case. It is possible to be sleep deprived as a senior citizen, something that goes unaddressed because of the myths circulating about sleep. We need sleep in order to rest, repair, and restore our system properly. (38), (39), (40)

Common Sleep Issues

Excessive sleepiness can be traced to a number of underlying problems, including sleep apnea and heart trouble. Getting regular checkups by the doctor can go a long way to better sleep.

You may recall that sleep apnea is a problem where your brain isn't getting oxygen at various intervals while you sleep. When your body is struggling for air, it creates sleep disruptions that leave you groggy the next day. Restless leg syndrome can also affect sleep cycles negatively; be sure to see your doctor to determine whether or not you have this condition.

Light is a major factor in sleep disruption, and most of us in this day and age are used to browsing Netflix on our phones, or on the TV now. Don't get me wrong; I love technology, and I think it really does benefit the world at large.

However, there are some negatives to technology, especially when it comes to health. It's very easy to slip into a state where we feel we need to catch that television episode, or we think that we can't go to sleep unless it's to a film.

The darker you can make your room, the better. Now, as we get older, sometimes our eyesight just isn't what it used to be. I'm not telling you to ignore common sense.

You can have small lights that you can touch and make your way to the bathroom safely. If you need to go down any flight of stairs, don't try to just feel your way through in the dark.

That might sound obvious, but you'd be surprised how many slip and fall accidents are caused by thinking you have more visibility than you do, especially at night. (41)

Make sure that you turn that television off, ditch the phone at least two hours before bed, and stay in a dark room. If your sleep still doesn't improve after a few weeks, it might be time to talk to your doctor about other treatment pathways they can try out.

So, to recap this chapter:

- Light is the enemy of good sleep everywhere. Minimize the lights in your bedroom as much as possible. If you or a loved one needs to get up and down during the middle of the night, use light to make a clear path to the restroom.
- Sleep apnea can become an underlying factor in poor sleep quality. If you suspect that you might be having intervals during sleep where you aren't breathing or sleep that just isn't giving you the energy you deserve, it's time to call the doctor. Don't skip this step; sleep apnea can be dangerous, and should be monitored under a doctor's careful eye.

HIIT Workout Time

Getting in shape, like most things in life, certainly isn't about following a straight line. I know from first-hand experience that it takes a lot longer than people may expect to get to the point where they're truly active on a regular basis.

I'm often stopped while running around my neighborhood and complimented about how great I look. People don't realize that even when you're coming from a fairly active background, life can have a way of making you slow down really quick.

When I was dealing with stressful classes at my university, I ate badly like everyone else I knew. I struggled with weight because I felt like no matter what I did, I just couldn't break the hold that my stress had on me.

Of course, this was a personal problem that I had to overcome to get back to the physique I wanted. But even after I decided to lose weight, it wasn't like the pounds just vanished overnight.

I had to get serious about how I was about to get started, and I didn't let anyone stand in my way from that point forward. I'm sure that a few people got their feelings hurt, but I knew that I needed to be take care of myself first and foremost. As the old saying goes, you can't serve anyone a cup of coffee if your own internal pot is empty.

Let's set down a proper foundation before we get to the actual fitness section. What I'm going to discuss in this part of the guide is all about high intensity interval training, known as HIIT.

Now, one person's HIIT framework is going to look very different from another person's framework, even though they're in the same category. The reason why is that HIIT responds well to your current fitness levels, while giving you the ability to move the intensity up or down based on your needs.

If things start getting easier, you can add more weight, more reps, or reduce the time allotted to the task. It's completely up to you, but there are plenty of ways to increase the difficulty that you're unlikely to get bored of this.

Now, if you're still working through the "Block by Block" walking challenge, this might not be a section that you can dive into right away.

But still read through it to get a good idea of what's waiting for you as things get easier walking around the neighborhood. I'll have you running and pushing your body to new heights soon enough!

What defines an HIIT workout? Well, it's any time that we do any type of exercise within a specific time period, as intensely as possible, and then follow it up with a rest period.

So if you wanted to try your hand at running but didn't want to put in six miles like I do, you could go the HIIT route.

You could jog for a minute, and then walk around the block for 2 minutes. That would be a three minute interval total.

If you repeated that interval ten times, it would be a 30 minute workout that could be nearly as intense as me running a full mile as fast as I could (on a safe track, of course).

A lot of people like HIIT because they're pressed for time, and you can get a lot out of the intervals. In fact, a researcher named Dr. Izumi Tabata did a great deal of investigating just how well intensity could affect athletic performance.

While Tabata workouts are indeed classified as HIIT moves, that doesn't mean that all HIIT is Tabata. (42), (43), (44), (45)

Dr. Tabata started out looking at the link between our aerobic and anaerobic systems of the body. If you're out of the loop on what those terms mean, don't worry. Aerobic energy system affects our every day "long term" activities, the things that we need to do for more than just a few minutes.

The aerobic system in the body is directly affected by how well we can use oxygen to fuel muscle movement. To turn this into a clear explanation, think back to the last time you had to go for a run in school.

Chances are good that you managed to go for a few minutes, and then you started getting winded really quickly.

Or imagine having to climb a tall flight of stairs to get to the fifth floor of an office building. The first set of stairs might be fine, but by the time you get to the fifth floor you're going to be pretty tired.

The only way to improve being "winded" is to work on improving the aerobic system to the point where you can use the energy efficiently. HIIT directly affects not just our aerobic energy, but our anaerobic energy as well.

So if our aerobic system is all about long term, then anaerobic energy would have to be about the short bursts of power.

Let's say that you're cornered by someone that is trying to get too close to you, and you have to get away. You might not have to run far, but you're going to need a quick burst of energy to escape.

The anaerobic side governs this type of energy, and we improve it through sprints and other forms of power training.

Some of that might be well out of scope for this guide, since most seniors aren't trying to become amateur athletes. But I can still take the best pieces of athletic training to change your health, and that's what this section is all about.

Going back to Dr. Tabata, the initial Tabata Protocol was done on an ergometer, a piece of machinery that most people don't have. The research subjects were divided into two groups, but both groups had to use the ergometer.

The first group only had to pedal at 70% of V02max, a measure of their total capacity, and they did this for a full hour. However, the second group didn't have it this easy.

They were required to go as hard as they could for 20 seconds, then they got to rest for ten seconds. This continued in a cycle for four minutes, and eight sets were completed in that timeframe.

There was one constant: time. Each group had to continue the workout for 5 days every week, for 6 weeks. They did an average of 20 minutes for every workout day. You might expect the second group to have terrible results, since they only worked out for 4 minutes.

The results were actually interesting for their time. The second group that had the intense effort got similar results to the first group, even though they had an hour. The Tabata Protocol was well received because of this interesting insight, and the fitness world has run with it ever since. (46), (47), (48)

Now, the original study had two test groups, but they were both young athletic men in their 20s. If you're going to do HIIT, you might have more of a steep curve to overcome. That doesn't mean that you can't get something out of it, naturally.

HIIT Benefits

Now, I didn't tell you all of that stuff above about Dr. Tabata to leave you hanging without any benefits of HIIT.

You can not only improve aerobic and anaerobic systems with HIIT, but you can also keep your body's metabolism working harder post-HIIT exercise for longer versus simple walking.

If you've ever looked into strength training, you'll find similar benefits there as well. We can burn fat a lot longer after HIIT than when we go for a long but casual walk. (49), (50)

Quick HIIT Supply List

If you're going to get into HIIT, you'll need a few supplies to get started. The first piece of equipment would have to be an interval timer. This isn't a basic stopwatch, but you can find interval timers very inexpensively now.

The timer will help you switch from work periods to rest periods, so you'll use it over and over again for a very long time. You'll also need a notebook and a pen to take notes on your progress. When I first got into HIIT, I thought that I'd remember everything. Guess what?

A few weeks later when I wanted to review the data, I couldn't remember much of anything. I've learned from that mistake a thousand times over, because I didn't know what I needed to tweak in order to improve my performance.

Today, I immediately go to my computer or to my notebook to jot down how well I did and what else I feel I need to work on. If things are getting too easy, then I also know that I need to adjust what I'm doing.

Now, the equipment you add to your list for HIIT can vary. What I'm outlining here are just some ideas, and the exercises in my guide will use everything I list. But you might want to add something different, and I'm perfectly okay with that.

In fact, if you didn't customize what you were doing I'd probably feel a bit insulted. Everything in this guide is designed to be like modeling clay in your hands. It's going to give you the ability to put the clay in the templates and then pop out cool shapes, but you can sculpt something completely wonderful that's based on your needs.

If you don't have a standard weight set, you'll need to get somewhere that has one. Most community gyms will have all of the weights and machines that you could ask for, and senior citizens often get a very nice discount on a new membership.

I also recommend a dip station; because dips really help you build upper body strength. I've noticed a lot of seniors that get back into fitness have decent lower body strength but struggle to pick things up. Improving that upper body isn't just something nice to think about; you should consider it a requirement. A toned body from head to toe is the goal here.

You also need to think about the type of clothes you want to wear while you do your workout. You're going to work up quite a sweat during HIIT, so it's to your advantage to get lightweight clothes.

You'll find a variety of exercise clothes, so the rest of it is just based on your own unique tastes. I like to have shorts in the summer and very warm clothing in the winter. Of course, if your winters are milder than mine, just consider yourself lucky and go from there!

Warm-Up Phase

While I did go over warm-up information during the "Redefining Mobility" chapter, it's important that you warm up before each workout. You're going to be working a lot harder than just walking around now, so it pays to keep those muscles in great shape.

The exercises below are best suited for your warm-up, though we're sure that you could sneak them into other places. For the time being, let's just focus on the warm-up phase.

Child's Pose

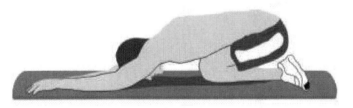

How to:

To pull off this move, you'll need to get down on your hands and knees. From here, you will want to move your knees until they're spread wide, but without breaking a connection between your feet. The big toe on each foot will need to connect to the other toe.

Now, from here, imagine becoming a long thin line on the floor. You need to begin to sit up, pulling your spine outward.

Take a deep breath, then as you exhale you'll want to tilt forward, putting your torso right between the tops of your thighs. The arms should be long, with your palms on the floor. Note that your head never really lifts from the ground.

Downward Dog

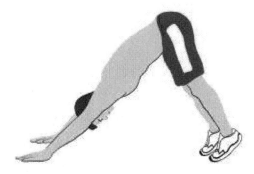

How to:

Most people mention this yoga pose first when anyone brings up the subject of yoga. Downward dog starts out as a standing pose and brings you down to the floor for the final position.

Start by getting on a good mat or just use the carpet on the floor. You need to start in the standing position, with your feet spread wide. From here, slowly lower yourself to the floor, but keeping your hips in the air.

Keep your hamstrings tight and your knees soft, avoiding pulling the tailbone in too far. Your back should be very straight as you move.

The weight will be resting on your hands, so make sure to keep them steady. Keep breathing through the entire pose!

Mountain Pose

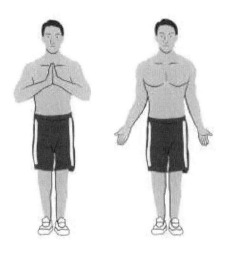

How to:

To start this move, you'll need to be standing tall and proud, with your feet pulled in tight. The arms need to be loose, completely opposite from the feet.

It might be tempting to let your shoulders and back slump or round, but try to avoid that part. Make sure that you put both of your big toes together and push your heels back. Lift the toes and then pull them apart slowly, moving one by one.

Push down through the heels to straighten your legs, full extension moving upward. You'll need to squeeze your legs together and rotate so your legs have a full stretch.

Chair Knee Extension

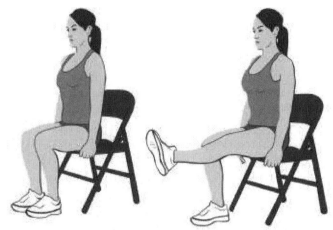

How to:

I love to include this warm-up stretch whenever I'm working with an older group. Sometimes if the idea of standing up to stretch is too much, this stretch is much easier to deal with until you can do harder moves.

In the middle of an active warm-up, the chair stretch is like a "break" without stopping the flow of activity. To get started, you'll need to sit towards the edge of a chair without risking falling from the seat.

Lift your right leg straight out, while keeping your left leg still. Once you have the right leg in position, lower it slowly to the floor. Your foot should be fully on the floor before you pause, and then switch things to the left leg.

Hamstring Stretch

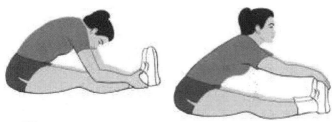

How to:
HIIT exercises are well known for using the whole body, so you want to make sure that your hamstrings are being prepped for the purpose.

You might not realize how many times a day your hamstrings engage to keep you stable, but they're pretty important! For this stretch, you'll need to get on the floor.

Take your right leg and tuck it in towards your belly-button, while leaving your left leg fully extended.

Lean forward so that you're turning towards your left leg and then move fully forward to pull on the hamstring gently. Keep things very light, smooth, and easy; I'm just looking for you to stretch. If things start burning, you've stretched too far and need to rest.

Toe Touch

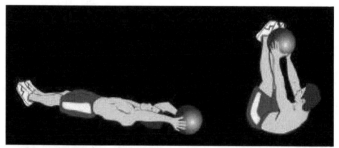

How to:

The toe touch is an easy move to pull off, but that doesn't mean that it's not important. You'll want to stretch fully because speed is going to be critical in the HIIT workouts you'll face.

If you aren't fully limber, you'll feel it the next day as your body struggles to compensate for the delays. To get this move started, you just need to get on the floor. Try to lay out as flat as possible, with your legs and arms fully extended.

At this point, all you have to do is bring your toes and hands together. They should be fully touching, and you'll need to hold this position for at least thirty seconds. After you hold the move for a few moments, let go and relax back at the starting position.

HIIT Exercise Library

This library is smaller than others, but don't underestimate it for a second! You'll want to get better at the exercises in this library before you mix things up.

All of these exercises can be done in an HIIT format as well as the traditional weight training style.

Even if we deviate from Dr. Tabata's protocol a bit, you can still get in a great workout session.

Be sure that you look carefully at all of the images for the technique, as well as my description of how to do everything. The last thing you want to do is injure yourself while you're just starting out.

Squat Jump

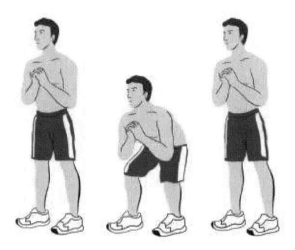

How to:

The squat jump is commonly referred to as an explosive move, and that lets you set yourself up for a really nice addition to your HIIT workout.

To get started with this move, you'll want to be standing straight up. Your feet should be about shoulder width apart, but not terribly wide.

You'll want to go into a full squat move, with your hips below parallel to the best of your ability. From this crouched down position, you'll want to push through your heels in order to spring back up to the starting position. You want to start standing and finish standing in order to complete one repetition.

Reverse Row

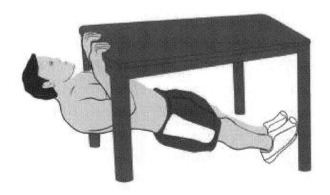

How to:

Do you want to improve your upper body strength? Look no further than the reverse row, since it builds on upper body strength and core strength at the same time. You'll need to use a good table or a chair in order to do the reverse row exercise.

To get started, get fully underneath the table with your hands firmly on the edge. You'll need this edge in order to pull yourself up to the top of the table.

You should be hanging by your hands with your feet on the floor, but your body turned on an invisible diagonal line. Pull yourself up to the ledge of the table, and then slowly drop back down. Try to avoid letting gravity do the work for you!

Frog Jump

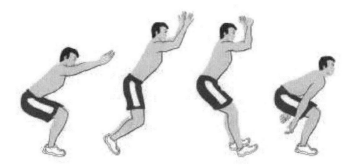

How to:

This is another explosive move I like, and it's good to get your blood moving in the morning! Start this move off right by getting into a semi-standing position. You can stand up, but get ready to crouch down and spring up again.

The feet should be wider than shoulder width apart, with the toes spread outward. Get into a deep squat, like you're stuck without a chair and you have to hunt something quietly.

From here, you need to jump as high as you can, while propelling yourself forward a little bit. This is like the squat jump but you've got a little distance mixed in, making it the frog jump instead. Think about how a frog moves, and you'll get the right idea.

One Legged Deadlift

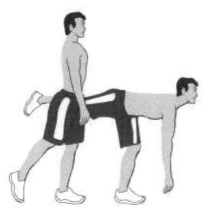

How to:

Didn't expect to see the word "deadlift" without seeing a barbell, right? Well, you can hold a dumbbell if you want but it's not necessary. You can do this move anywhere, and some people even add it to their warm-up to get really charged up before the day begins.

Since we're going to do it as part of our HIIT workout, we don't need to add it to anything else. Pulling off this move couldn't be easier: you just need to start with a standing position, with your left leg pushed half a stride behind you.

Your right leg should be straight, with your right foot placed firmly on the floor.

Keep your back arched just slightly, and your core muscles engaged. You have to be able to keep your body steady, and the core is a big part of that.

At this point, you'll want to tilt forward while pushing the hips back. Your hand should go parallel with the floor, without touching it. Hold this position for a few moments, then slowly use your back and core to get back to the starting position.

While it might be tempting, don't let gravity steal your results. If you let gravity do the work, you will not be able to get the same effect compared with doing the work yourself.

Good Mornings

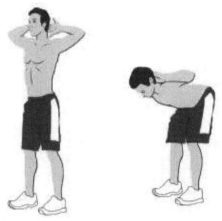

How to:

Despite the name of this exercise, good mornings are a great addition to your workout routine at any time of the day or night! This exercise uses the muscles of your back, making for a very intense HIIT addition.

Be sure that you aren't trying to get "more" out of the move by hyperextending the back. While speed is important, you should protect yourself by limiting the range of motion.

Start the move by getting into a standing position with your feet very wide apart. Bend your knees just a little bit, with your hands placed behind the head. Tilt your body forward from the hips, pushing your shoulders parallel to the floor.

The chest is how you'll know where to stop; it should be held parallel to the floor but nothing past that. After a few moments, slowly reverse tilt your body back to the starting position.

Reverse Lunge Swings

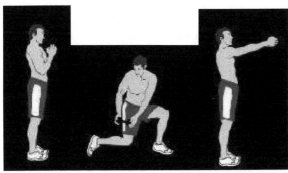

How to:

For this exercise, you'll need to have a pair of dumbbells. I recommend starting with a lighter set until you get the feel of this exercise.

Doing things in HIIT format means that there's a higher chance of injury if you're taking on weights that you really can't handle very well. To get started, take a single dumbbell into your hands, with each hand firmly holding the end of the dumbbell.

Get down into a classic lunge position, turning your body towards the bent side. If you start from the right, then you would be "turning" towards the left.

You'll want to swing from the down position back upward to your starting position in a clean, fluid motion. Pay very close attention to the dumbbell, as you don't want to let it fly out of your hands.

Dumbbell Thrusters

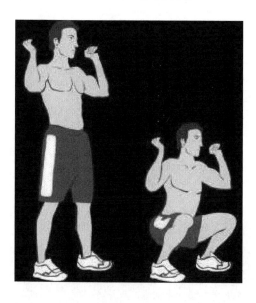

How to:

Longtime fans of my books will probably laugh at me for including dumbbell thrusters again. I like the exercise and add it to so many routines because it works multiple muscle groups, like your deltoids, biceps, and triceps.

So if you want to really improve upper body strength, thrusters are the way to go. Doing them right means that you pay attention to the little details as you go along. When you're ready to start this exercise, you'll need to stand up straight and proud while holding a dumbbell in each hand.

Lift them up so that they are parallel to your shoulders and then squat down until your hips are below your knees. Drive up by pushing through the heels and return back to the starting position, ensuring that the dumbbells aren't moving around wildly.

Standing Dumbbell Curl

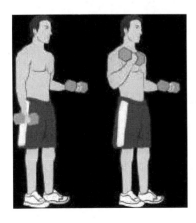

How to:

This exercise is another timeless favorite of mine. Every time I perform it, I definitely feel the muscles in my arms getting to work. You'll notice it too when you pull off the move. To get started, you'll need to grab a pair of your favorite dumbbells.

This is going to be the pair that is still challenging, but not so much that you're straining to pick them up. Shift your arms in order to turn your palms forward-facing. Bend your elbows and curl the dumbbells in as close as possible, all without moving the upper arms. Take a few moments, and then go back to the starting position.

Mountain Climbers

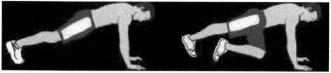

How to:

The mountain climber move is challenging but fun; it just takes some time to get used to doing it regularly. To get started, you want to get into push-up position, with your hands and feet on the floor.

From this point, you will pull your left leg into a "step" position, like you're about to climb either a flight of stairs slowly or the side of a mountain.

Hold the left leg in the air for a moment, then bring it back down, quickly switching over to the right leg.

Repeat the process for the right leg, and then go back to the starting position. As you might imagine from the images below, this is quite the workout move when done in HIIT format. Try it out!

Dumbbell Lunge

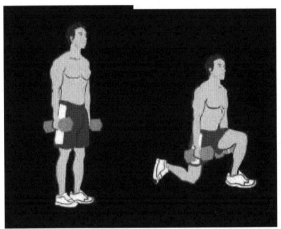

How to:

Break out your dumbbells, because I'm about to introduce another move that'll require a set of weights. The dumbbell lunge is all about precise control. You don't want to let gravity get in the way of your workout at any time or for any reason.

But once you see how easy it is to pull off the move, you won't want to turn to gravity anyway. Get started by standing up straight with a dumbbell in each hand. Your arms should rest loosely at your sides, and your core should already be tight.

Take one step forward, almost like you were striding across a great desert step by step. Most people like to step out on the right leg first, then the left leg. If you follow that pattern, you'll step with the right leg, forming an angle slightly greater than 90 degrees.

Your left leg will bend down to a little less than 90 degrees, with the knee hovering just above the floor. Hold this position, and then slowly use your core and legs to go back to the starting position.

Dip

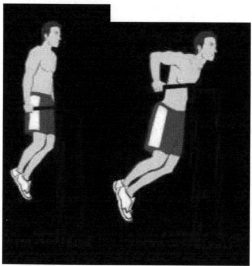

How to:
I hesitate sometimes to include the dip, because it's a move that tends to frustrate people.

While it seems simple on paper, doing it in real time becomes a different story. It's better to make sure that you learn how to do this exercise properly. The dip I'm focusing on is the triceps dip, which not only targets those triceps, but also your deltoids as well.

Let's get started by approaching the dip station. You want to place your hands on the dip station securely, keeping those hands in line with your shoulders. Your legs have to be extended fully with the knees only slightly bent. From here, just lower yourself down until your shoulders "dip" below the elbow from the top. Hold for a moment, and then push upward until you're back to the starting position.

Standing Pike Crunch

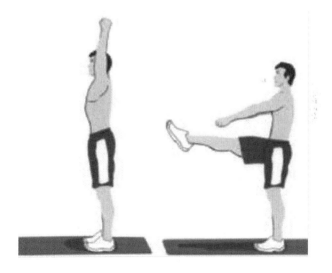

How to:

The standing pike crunch is a great way to add some fun back into crunches. Most people think of the crunch only as something you have to do on the floor, but that's not the case at all here. Not only will you start in a standing position, you'll finish there as well. No, really, check it out: you start by standing tall with your knees just slightly bent.

Get ready to move fast, because you'll need to bring your right foot up and connect it back to your right hand. Don't swing or let gravity do the job; just make it a fluid movement with your leg.

Keep the core muscles tight as you bring the foot upward, and then move back to the starting position. You'll switch legs, and do it again before it's all said and done.

7 Day Workout Cycle

I recommend that you start with 15 minute workouts. Between the walking you're already doing and these workouts, you're set up for great fat loss. Don't be surprised if you find that your body looks very different in the mirror after a month or two.

The way the 15 minute session will work is like this: you'll do one minute of effort for each exercise, then 2 minutes of rest. Since you're moving as intensely as possible during that minute, you'll definitely be glad that you can rest for 2 minutes afterward.

This is also why the interval timer is so important, because you can adjust it to meet your needs. Once the timer sounds the end of the rest period, you'll need to get back to work.

This is a 7 day cycle with three workout days, and four rest days. Now, you will not start working intensely until you've gotten the basic workout under your belt. The goal here is to gradually work your way up into more fitness. If you rush into a super intense workout schedule from the beginning, you'll burn out before you get to really see what your body can do.

Monday

Warm-Up Phase (reference the warm-up exercises above)

15 minute session - Each exercise should be done in a 1 minute work / 2 minutes rest format
- Squat Jump
- Frog Jump
- Dumbbell Thrusters
- Mountain Climbers
- Dip

Tuesday

Rest day

See how you're feeling so far! You can go for a light walk, get some cleaning done around the house, or just prep your meals for the next few days. If you're really feeling sore, don't worry. Some soreness is indeed normal.

You're going from a more sedentary lifestyle to being active, and it could take a few months before you're truly well-adjusted. But every journey starts with this initial period of soreness. You might feel like nothing is happening, but the benefits will accumulate well over time. Just hang in there!

Wednesday

Warm-Up Phase (reference the warm-up exercises above)

15 minute session - Each exercise should be done in a 1 minute work / 2 minutes rest format
- Dumbbell Thrusters
- Dumbbell Lunge
- Standing Pike Crunch
- Standing Dumbbell Curl
- Dip

Thursday

Rest day

You're doing great! Why not take today to update all of your tracking? As I mentioned earlier in this guide, tracking your results from the beginning gives you a rich treasure trove of data to sift through later on in your journey.

I like to review my progress week to week, especially when I'm restarting a fitness plan. Hey, I'm human and even I can get distracted from my goals. You can always go for a walk today. Have you updated your progress on the Block by Block walking challenge?

This would be a great day to add some miles to your total walking distance. The worst thing you could do is just sit on the couch all day, especially when you'll want to do a workout session tomorrow.

Friday

Warm-Up Phase (reference the warm-up exercises above)

15 minute session - Each exercise should be done in a 1 minute work / 2 minutes rest format

- Reverse Row
- One Legged Deadlift
- Good Mornings
- Reverse Lunge Swing
- Squat Jump

Saturday & Sunday

Rest Days

Follow the same tips from the other rest days. You can even relax completely. Making time for friends and family is good when you're entering a new workout cycle. They should be happy that you're getting more active.

Improving your longevity through exercise might be long term, but over time your family will notice some subtle differences. They may notice that you don't get winded when you go up a flight of steps, or when you have to bend down to get something from the floor.

They may compliment you when they notice that your clothes hang differently, or that you have to go shop for new clothes to wear.

A rest day should be a break for the mind as well as the body. Indulging in a good book while the weather is breezy and calm is never a bad idea, and you can always get right back into the swing of things on your workout days.

Evaluating Your Workout

So, after your first week you'll want to look at your progress. Don't assume that you're automatically in for a rough time. You can do this! Each week will get easier and easier.

Yes, I know I'm repeating myself a bit. Believe me, for people that are just starting out, they need the reminder as much as they can hear it.

If you're coming into this at a more advanced level, there's a chance that you won't be challenged that much. There are ways to remedy this problem, from increasing the intensity of your workout to adding more weight to the weighted exercises.

You could also increase the number of intervals you're doing for each session. It's very easy to make a 30 minute workout instead of a 15 or a 20 minute workout if you're trying to take things a bit slower.

If you want to take away a rest day, you can definitely do that. Remember that Saturday and Sunday are automatically rest days here. Perhaps instead of a full on HIIT workout, you want to add in something else? You could lift weights on one of those days, or go for a longer walk than you usually do.

There are other questions that you'll need to answer on your journey, and writing the answers down in your official fitness and food log will help you remember them over time.

You want to ask yourself if the workouts are really too easy, or if you're skipping good form in the name of speed.

Never sacrifice form, because you invite a greater risk of injury if you do. You also want to see if adding another intensity day is really the best thing to do. If you're someone that knows you can handle it, jump in and see what you can do. You can always go back down to three workouts if things get a little too intense.

Post-Workout Tips

One of the first things that people ask about when it comes to post-workout tips is whether or not they should go home and eat. If you find that you're hungry, by all means...go and eat!

Obviously, if you're going to eat something it should be on your blueprint.

Don't ruin your hard work by hitting up the closest fast food place. While they may have an inexpensive menu, you can get nourishing food from the store that you packed ahead of time.

It's true that we're all busier than we've ever been, but I have seen plenty of people prepare to go to the gym.

Treat it like going somewhere important where you're going to have to have certain items in order to complete the task.

Would you go there without an important file? Even if you were just doing something as mild as going to the grocery store, would you leave your house without your shopping list? You could do that, of course, but there are obvious consequences to consider.

I like to eat a great deal of food after I return from a good workout session. However, I only eat until I'm somewhat full.

By the time I've finished a big glass of water, I just don't feel like packing in any more food. It can take a long time to get to this point, and you might feel frustrated that you're not here yet.

However, the truth of the matter is that you could have your hormones working against you right now, blocking your weight loss. Thankfully there are solutions to this problem.

What problem might be lurking in the shadows, keeping you from the weight loss that you want? Leptin resistance.

Most people have never heard of leptin, and they still don't think that it can do anything to them. You may be surprised.

Hunger in the body is controlled by leptin, a hormone that signals to the brain not only when you're hungry, but your energy levels as a whole.

Keeping the human body from starving used to be a full time job. While things have changed in our society due to technology, leptin didn't get this memo.

So it still works around the clock to keep you from starving, even though it's mostly unnecessary. We have more food than we really know what to do with, and so overeating is more of a problem than eating too little. (51), (52)

When leptin goes wrong, it doesn't signal the brain properly. This means that our loyal hormone doesn't actually go back to telling the brain that we are doing okay and don't need to store all of this fat.

Considering that fat cells are direct producers of leptin, you can start to see just how crazy things get when leptin resistance is in full swing.

Why am I talking about leptin and leptin resistance in the fitness section of this book? Because we can turn things around for the better through exercise, of course!

Leptin levels are lowered through physical activity, and HIIT activities play a great role in lowering leptin resistance.

Eating protein will also help, as it tends to improve how well leptin communicates with the brain. This is often referred to as leptin sensitivity.

Since you're committing to less processed food as part of your new eating habits and framework, you're already on track to making broken leptin levels a thing of the past.

Is good eating just about dodging leptin? Not at all! Getting a good night's sleep is equally important, so be sure that you're taking care of both needs.

Lowering your stress will also help you decrease the amount of leptin encouraging your body to not only hold onto the pounds you already have, but pack on more pounds to keep you going.

Like most things in your new lifestyle, it's all about balancing what you eat, how active you are, and how well you sleep. If one of those things begins to fall out of balance, the entire system will fall apart before you know it.

After you work out, you'll want to track not only the meal you just ate, but the activities that led you to get hungry in the first place. If you worked out in a gym, then you'll want to record all of those exercises.

Later, when you review all of this data, you may be able to spot patterns that will either help you improve, or at least give you something to work on.

There could be advances and progress points that you want to savor, and I believe these are as important as identifying the challenges ahead of time. If you don't celebrate, you'll get discouraged.

So, to recap this chapter:

- Working out is a great deal for the heart and body, but it also makes us feel better on the inside. Lowering the potential for depression is never a bad thing!
- Choose good workout gear for every session, because items that are too tight or too baggy can interfere with movement.
- It cannot be stressed enough: wear good shoes all the time, even when you feel like you want to take them off and go barefoot. Shoes are designed to protect the foot, but you might need to try on a few pairs before you really find what you're looking for.
- Setting up your first HIIT session might cost you a little bit upfront, but it'll pay off for many years to come.
- Don't force any HIIT move; your first few rounds may not be the best, but they'll get better.
- Repeat the 7 day cycle for a period of 4 weeks, and then evaluate your progress. What are you really good at? What do you need to work on?
- Tracking fitness and food together can help you spot patterns that may have otherwise been overlooked.

Overcoming Obstacles

Every lifestyle change has its fair share of speed bumps, things that come up along the way that throw you off. The more I talk about health, the more people pull up a chair to listen.

Somewhere after my 20th book I realized that people were starting to take their health seriously but still had some questions come up. Now, you might wonder why people didn't just tell me outright that a lot of the things I was talking about and teaching just weren't working for them.

It's simple: pride. In other words, it's hard for people to come clean when they fear that they're going to be rejected. It's not necessarily that I rejected them, but that they are used to people telling them that they are too ambitious, that they want more than what they deserve.

Folks, I fully believe that better health can be around the corner for you. Does that mean it will be virtually overnight?

Not at all.

Depending on where you're starting from, the road to good health could be miles and miles down the highway. You have to be willing to face that as you look closer at how things are going.

I'll cover some classic problems that come up, along with some suggestions to try out. Since all of this is experimentation and based on unique circumstances, you may have to try multiple solutions before things even themselves out.

Low Energy

Low energy is something that a lot of people struggle with, even before they make a lifestyle change. So it can be extremely frustrating to be on a plan and not get the boost in energy that you were looking for.

Energy balance is a pretty complicated topic, and whole books are dedicated to this subject alone. I can tell you that if you're struggling with low energy, you're certainly not struggling with it by yourself.

Plenty of people shift to a low carb diet, and there's a transitioning period where you're going to feel a bit strange while your body adapts to running primarily on fat first and carbs second. It's this transition that often triggers a very fatigued feeling, but it generally goes away in a few weeks.

In the meantime, taking B-12 supplements (preferably methylcobalamin-based ones) can help you with raising your energy levels. It is also important that you really avoid the sweets during this initial period, so your body doesn't try to go back to running primarily off of carbohydrates.

Leg Cramps

Generally speaking, leg cramps could be from getting used to working out, or they can be linked to low levels of magnesium in your diet. By tracking your food regularly, you'll be able to go back and see how much magnesium you're getting in the day's meals.

It's easy to imagine getting enough magnesium, until you realize that this is a vital mineral in the body that is easily depleted day by day. We have to continually get magnesium in order to live, and leg cramps can be a sign that your levels are really low.

If your leg cramps are eased through warm compresses and rest, it could be a sign that you've just pushed too hard in the gym and it's time to add another rest day to your plan.

Don't feel discouraged if you have to go from doing three workouts to two, or if you've recently increased the intensity of your workouts and now you're looking at scaling back. Everyone goes through a phase where they have to make a lot of adjustments in order to really get in the swing of things.

Constipation

Even though you've moved your food choices around, you still require a few things in order to maintain your health.

If you're dealing with constipation or other digestive issues, you really need to consider adding more fiber sources to your diet. I'm aware that I cautioned against oats, rice, and other high carb foods.

However, those aren't the only foods that can help you increase your fiber intake every day. The classic ingredients of a salad will provide a good source of fiber, as well as much needed variety in your diet.

In fact, most vegetables give you plenty of fiber and there are lots of low carb options. I like cauliflower, cabbage, broccoli, and spaghetti squash the most.

No Weight Loss

If you're struggling with the scale right now, you certainly have my sympathies. There are few things are stressful as going through the steps to change your lifestyle and still not seeing the scale reflect any changes.

Yet there's more to this picture than meets the eye, and not studying things carefully can lead you to believe that nothing is happening. When you take on a fitness and diet change, you're changing things from the inside out.

You really do have to think about this as a journey that will take time. So the scale might not be moving, but are there other signs of progress? Can you lift things that you couldn't lift before?

Do you notice that your dumbbells have gotten heavier, or that you can do more intense fitness intervals than before? Are your clothes fitting better, or have you gotten to shop around for new clothes? These are valid changes and they're more important than the numbers on the scale. Why?

That's easy: it reflects that your life is moving in a positive direction. When people come to me anxious about their progress, I like to remind them that they are just getting started.

Don't panic if you don't see big changes within a month after giving this framework your best efforts. Start looking for more visible signs of progress at the 3-4 month mark.

Weight Gain

Gaining weight after changing your lifestyle is the last thing that anyone wants to think about. However, the stress of life can cause us to veer away from the things that we really want to do. If you're struggling with weight gain, there are two main causes: environment and bad habits.

Stress can be a product of the environment that you have to work with, but there are ways to deal with that. Sometimes it might mean that you have to set new boundaries with the people that you interact with on a regular basis, or you may need to change other elements of your environment.

I have a dear friend that could only focus on her needs after she went through a very painful and prolonged divorce. While the divorce was very difficult, she could finally focus on fitness activities without her former spouse making her feel guilty for needing time for her own hobbies.

As far as eating habits go, there are adjustments that you might need to make here. If you've taken the time to carefully track everything that you've eaten, as well as the drinks you've enjoyed. Soda can be very sneaky and hide not only calories, but plenty of sugar.

You also want to look at drinks mixed with alcohol, because sweetened liquors can still carry carbs that we didn't expect. If you absolutely must have alcohol, you'll need to focus on liquors rather than mixed drinks.

Liquors like whiskey and vodka have zero carbs, making them perfect for seltzer and sugar-free sweeteners and syrups. When I'm really working on my body, I avoid alcohol most of the time.

Sure, there's a celebration here and there, but my focus is on staying in good shape. It's very easy to enjoy a toast at one wedding and then find yourself pouring a small glass every night. All of those drinks add up, and not in a way that improves performance.

At the end of the day, you have to base all of your decisions on one question: is it going to improve my performance, or take away from what I've worked very hard to get? That's the most important question, and only you can answer it.

Feeling Hungry

A lot of people that really get into HIIT report that they're hungrier than ever before. And because they're so used to broken eating habits that don't serve them, they just assume that all hunger types are bad. Most people haven't been overeating in the past because they were suffering from severe hunger.

Our society as a whole has access to more food than it really knows what to do with. The difference is that we've turned food into an entertainment, as well as a way to avoid confronting certain issues or feelings.

If you're eating junk food because you're reeling from a family tragedy, it's understandable. But sooner or later, you'll have to remember what your goals are and how good you're going to feel as you reach different milestones.

One of the people I admire is Ernestine Shepherd, who currently holds record for being the world's oldest female bodybuilder. She decided to walk down that path after losing her sister, and she's never looked back.

Her body reflects several years of hard work and overcoming challenges. She's in her 70s and is still getting up every day to do the work.

When I start feeling sorry for myself, I remember that I still have a lot of family that checks on me, and I have enough health to get up and do the work...just like Ms. Shepherd does every day.

These problems can be overcome, and I believe that good solutions could be lurking right under your nose. Don't just read these suggestions and think that they don't apply to you.

Unless your doctor has you on a different treatment program or has warned you against taking a certain supplement, you owe it to yourself to try whatever it takes to feel better.

So, to recap this chapter:

- Be sure that you take these "obstacles" seriously. For example, you may dismiss thirstiness as just part of life, but it could be a sign that you're not getting enough fluids.

- If you've been really loose with your eating, it's time to get back on track. The only person that can confirm or deny this is the person looking back at you in the mirror. Even if you're logging everything perfectly, you may be underestimating another food or forgetting to put it in your log. Being completely honest about your eating habits will give you the best quality in terms of what data you can collect.

- Immediately inform your doctor if you become dizzy or extremely nauseated as a result of starting an exercise program, and follow their guidelines. Stay safe!

- Do not stop taking any medication until a doctor gives you their approval. While it's true that your new lifestyle may change how much medication you require, the only person that can help you determine that is a licensed medical professional.
- Too many flex days? Try to keep the junk away by turning to more fat sources. Fat is very satisfying, and it doesn't take much before you're full.

Taking Consistent Action

What's the missing ingredient that will form a bridge between the knowledge in this book and your goals? Why, action of course! You have to take consistent action in order to get from one side of the equation to the other.

Unfortunately, when friends walk up to me to discuss their fitness goals, I find myself having to hear their frustration that things haven't really taken off just yet. These are younger people, but the fun thing about fitness is that it really isn't as "age specific" as people think.

The body loves to be put to work, and improves the more that we put the body through its paces. Seniors have extra challenges due to the fact that they most likely have decades of inactivity to contend with, but you can improve your body over time.

Consistency is not just about setting the initial goal, but also following through with that goal no matter how hard it gets. Does that mean throwing yourself into a workout every day? Not at all.

When I advise people to be consistent, I'm telling them not to look for results on day 1, or 7, or 14, or 30.

I'm asking people to stay the course for as long as it takes. When you first get started on this framework, chances are good that you're going to secretly hope for fast changes.

I'm not picking on you; that's just the basic reality of human nature. We're all secretly looking for the fastest way to get what we want, and an entire industry has popped up to give people what they believe they want.

There is no "fast lane" to weight loss, but there are things that we can do in order to jumpstart the process. By changing your eating habits, you're taking the biggest step necessary in changing your health for the better.

Below, I'll break down three main areas where consistent action is necessary to pull off the framework properly.

I'm basing a lot of the information here from reports I've received from seniors that I got to meet face to face and guide them on this framework.

If you're looking to get started quickly and on the right track, this chapter is definitely one to look into.

Food

Managing food traditions is just one aspect of being consistent when it comes to food. The other part is making sure that you set up your meals in advance.

Giving yourself time to prepare your meals will play a big role in keeping you away from the type of food that helped weaken your health in the first place. Does that mean that you'll never have ice cream again?

Not at all.

There are sugar-free varieties of the treats we love, but we have to get to a point where we're not ruled by those treats. It's more important to avoid overdoing the "free treats", especially if you don't have a good hold over your eating habits.

If you want to get started on the right track from the start, you have to immediately get rid of the food that doesn't fit your framework. Some people do well with Flex days, where they can add in things like sweet potatoes or a heaping cup of rice.

Other people aren't going to be able to handle the Flex days, and will need to stick to the Focus days where everything is not only on plan but measured. If it isn't second nature to measure and weigh everything before you log it in your book, you'll get there.

If you want to be consistent, then you have to build clean data to work with from the beginning. Tracking your food will give you a lot of insight into other things, like the core of your habits.

If you tend to eat because you're bored, your logs will ultimately reveal that. Have a tendency to crave snacks during the day?

There's nothing wrong with eating some cut up veggies and cottage cheese to take the edge off your hunger. Stay the course!

Fitness

Working out regularly is something that people know they need to do, but it often goes to the bottom of our daily task list.

We have so many different demands playing on our time that we don't know where to begin. Instead of waiting till the end of the day to work out, why not make it one of the first things that you do?

The truth about fitness is that you'll only improve if you set out to make it a priority. I run in the morning because I know I have a full day on my plate.

I'd rather run and come to my to-do list ready for the events of the day than approach running at the end of the day when I'm just ready to unwind and get ready for bed.

HIIT workouts aren't for everyone, but there are ways to get your body in better condition while you ease into it. Walking is a great way to break the ice, because you can increase the intensity.

It's the difference between a casual walk where you're just enjoying the sight of the flowers, and a brisk walk where you have very little time to even sing along with music, let alone have a conversation with your walking buddy.

The best advice I can give here is to make sure that you start sooner than later. The body rewards ongoing activity with better conditioning, which is what we really need to enjoy the very short life that we're given.

Work through the fitness moves until they become second nature; you won't regret it for an instant.

Sure, you might have some aches and pains the next day for a while, but it'll get better.

If you're lacking the motivation to work out because you're alone, why not join a group? Fitness groups aren't just for "the young ones"; there are groups for the young at heart as well.

Now, a lot of younger people aren't prickly at the idea of older people working out right next to them.

But I will admit that there are just topics that are much more understandable when discussed with someone that's already put in a lot of years on this planet.

The stories that most of the senior citizens I've met have to tell blow me away, but their friends wouldn't really consider it all that earth-shattering.

After all, they have similar stories to share. My point is simple: go where you're celebrated, welcomed, and cherished.

This idea makes sense where I'm talking about community gyms or a meet-up for seniors in the community. Always go where you're celebrated, not chased away.

Lifestyle

If you're already changing your food habits and your fitness habits, the only thing that's left is to change your lifestyle habits.

A lifestyle covers a broad range of habits, but it's important to be very self-aware in terms of how the habits you have affect your progress.

For example, are you currently a smoker? Some people have smoked for a very long time and are very aware of the damage they're doing to their bodies.

If you're an active smoker, working out is going to be tougher because HIIT demands a lot of your lungs. You're testing your cardiovascular system to its limits, and smoking affects your ability to do that well.

Quitting smoking takes effort, and I'm the last person to tell you that it's easy. I never got into a serious smoking habit, but I've known people that do smoke and seeing them puff away on those cigarettes makes me pretty sad.

You have to examine all of the reasons you personally have to quit and then take action by replacing your smoking time with productive time. Believe it or not, smokers spend a lot of hours every year just in the act of using tobacco.

There are tons of support groups decided to not just weight loss, but ending smoking habits. Sometimes you can even find a group that handles both topics very well. If you are going to get into a group, go in with a service-led mind.

In other words, you'll get taken care of as long as you're willing to take care of someone else. This develops the strong community bonds that make support groups worthwhile in the first place.

Stress management plays a heavy role in how well we sleep and how much we get out of our fitness routine. If the body is already under great stress, working out is only going to make it worse.

But if we focus on working out mindfully where we're respecting our own natural boundaries, you can only improve over time.

Don't expect miracles from the very first day. You may have to deal with family issues, like losing a loved one or seeing a long-time friend have to be transferred into long term care.

That's never easy to deal with, but it is part of life. Growing older means not just getting bolder, but truly aging. We're not as young as we used to be, and time truly is fleeting.

Don't hold grudges when it's much easier to hold hands and forgive the slights found sometimes in day to day conversation. Anger only makes it harder to see your long-term goals.

Write down your real goals beyond just losing weight. Perhaps you've dreamed about being able to play in the park with the grandkids, rather than sitting on the bench like you've always done.

Maybe you want to set a better example to the nieces and nephews that grew up, but they're still watching every move you make. Fighting obesity is important at every age and in society at large.

You never know how deeply you inspire someone until you see them transform before your eyes. Naturally, everyone's a little vain on the inside.

It's totally fine that you imagine how good you could look if you were to lose some weight. My hope is just that you'll build some other goals along the way.

So, to recap this chapter:

- Give yourself the chance to succeed! Taking action from the beginning means that you're much more likely to stay the course.
- Do you feel discouraged when you first start out on something new? Joining a support group where you can be held accountable and also help other seniors feel accountable would be a wise idea.
- Don't let other people's opinions get in your head. If they aren't working on their health, why does their opinion really matter to you?

The Road Ahead

If you don't get any other message from this book, take this one with you: no one in the world has more ability to change your health than you do. The authority is in your hands, and should always stay there. Unfortunately, the world doesn't always work that way.

We've been programmed as a society to chase one get-thin-quick scheme after another, and our health has suffered in the process. There's a better way, but it does require commitment. Yes, I'm the commitment guy telling you that not only can you improve, but you can do the work as well.

Most things in life are expanded as long as we're willing to do the work necessary to go where we wish to truly live. If you want to live in the realm of improved health, you have to take the steps.

I've given you some additional tips, laid out a fitness framework and a food framework as well. I've talked about improving your sleep, and letting go of toxic relationships that bring nothing but stress to the table.

But here, I turn the microphone back over to you. It's your life and the choices you make will determine the road ahead. If you approach the information with an eagerness to get started, I only see good things ahead for you.

That's all I ask. Don't let this book be another one that collects dust in your collection, read only once and abandoned in hopes of the next book that tells you where the real health gold lives.

Friends, the potential for vibrant and amazing health is your birthright. It's our present for being human, and it's high time that all of us start prizing better health as a priority.

We can do a lot of things in this world, but we can't turn back time. Don't beat yourself up if you're just taking steps now to improve your health. Sometimes I have moments where I'm not thrilled to be out running, but I run because I know it benefits me in the long run. You will find yourself thinking similar thoughts as you begin your journey.

I truly appreciate everyone reading this guide, and I hope that you've gained more than just a few nuggets of wisdom from these pages. Take the first few wobbly steps to a new lifestyle and the benefits can be beyond your wildest imagination.

Even if there are stumbles along the way, know that you're walking a journey than millions of other people have taken. It's been the consistent ones, the determined ones, and the driven ones that made it to not just the end of their goals, but a life they truly cherish inside and out.

May you find what you seek on your journey.

All the best,

Mirsad Hasic

References

1. http://healthland.time.com/2012/08/29/want-to-live-longer-dont-try-caloric-restriction/

2.http://main.poliquingroup.com/ArticlesMultimedia/Articles/Article/1069/Ten _Amazing_Benefits_of_Eating_Fat.aspx

3. http://www.westonaprice.org/know-your-fats/the-importance-of-saturated-fats-for-biological-functions/

4. http://www.westonaprice.org/know-your-fats/the-importance-of-saturated-fats-for-biological-functions/

5. http://blog.ketoship.com/2016/02/26/the-best-healthy-fats-low-carb-diet/

6. http://www.huffingtonpost.ca/dr-mike-hart/saturated-fats_b_3641895.html

7. http://time.com/2863227/ending-the-war-on-fat/

8. http://articles.mercola.com/sites/articles/archive/2013/01/16/cholesterol-regulates-cell-signaling.aspx

9. http://www.thankyourbody.com/vegetable-oils/

10. https://authoritynutrition.com/6-reasons-why-vegetable-oils-are-toxic/

11. https://authoritynutrition.com/optimize-omega-6-omega-3-ratio/

12. http://www.hsph.harvard.edu/nutritionsource/what-should-you-eat/protein/

13. http://ajcn.nutrition.org/content/87/5/1558S.long

14. https://www.bulletproofexec.com/bulletproof-editorial-for-the-new-york-times-why-eating-meat-is-ethical/

15. http://lowcarbdiets.about.com/od/nutrition/p/fiberinfo.htm

16. http://ultimatepaleoguide.com/dairy/

17. http://www.webmd.com/diet/6-reasons-to-get-your-diary

18. http://www.paleoplan.com/2011/12-07/dairy-is-not-paleo/

19. https://authoritynutrition.com/6-ways-wheat-can-destroy-your-health/

20. http://wellnessmama.com/575/problem-with-grains/

21. http://www.marksdailyapple.com/are-oats-healthy/

22. http://www.whfoods.com/genpage.php?tname=foodspice&dbid=48

23. http://www.cbsnews.com/news/daily-tracking-could-improve-weight-loss/

24. http://nihseniorhealth.gov/falls/bonehealth/01.html

25. https://www.nlm.nih.gov/medlineplus/seniorshealth.html

26. https://health.clevelandclinic.org/2014/05/supplements-taking-many-can-hurt/

27. http://www.drweil.com/drw/u/QAA293439/How-Much-Calcium-is-Too-Much.html

28. http://umm.edu/health/medical/altmed/supplement/magnesium

29. http://ods.od.nih.gov/factsheets/VitaminA-HealthProfessional/

30.http://www.niams.nih.gov/Health_Info/Bone/Bone_Health/Nutrition/vitamin_a.asp

31. http://ods.od.nih.gov/factsheets/VitaminD-HealthProfessional/

32. http://articles.chicagotribune.com/2011-10-26/news/ct-x-1026-health-briefs-20111026_1_vitamin-d-deficiency-skin-sun-exposure

33. http://www.drweil.com/drw/u/ART02804/vitamin-k.html

34. http://www.health.harvard.edu/blog/two-questions-can-reveal-mobility-problems-in-seniors-201309186682

35. http://mashable.com/2011/05/09/sitting-down-infographic/

36. http://www.mayoclinic.org/healthy-lifestyle/fitness/in-depth/walking/art-20046261

37. http://www.unm.edu/~lkravitz/Article%20folder/musclesgrowLK.html

38. http://www.webmd.com/sleep-disorders/features/do-seniors-need-less-sleep

39. http://nihseniorhealth.gov/sleepandaging/aboutsleep/01.html

40. http://seniors.lovetoknow.com/Sleep_Apnea_in_Elderly

41. https://sleepfoundation.org/ask-the-expert/electronics-the-bedroom

42. http://www.acefitness.org/acefit/healthy-living-article/60/104/what-is-high-intensity-interval-training-hiit/

43. http://blog.fitsessions.com.au/2015/05/12/hiitvslissforcardio/

44. http://www.senior-exercise-central.com/The_Gray_Iron_Fitness_Newsletter-high-intensity-intervals.html

45.http://fitness.mercola.com/sites/fitness/archive/2013/04/12/tabata-workout.aspx

46.http://sportsmedicine.about.com/od/anatomyandphysiology/a/VO2_max.htm

47.http://journals.lww.com/acsm-healthfitness/Fulltext/2014/09000/TABATA__It_s_a_HIIT_.6.aspx

48. http://www.bodybuilding.com/fun/ask-the-ripped-dude-hiit.html

49. http://anthonycolpo.com/how-good-is-hiit-for-fat-loss-really/

50. http://www.gugly.com/Archswimaerobic.htm

51. http://www.ncbi.nlm.nih.gov/pmc/articles/PMC3281561/

52. http://wellnessmama.com/5356/fix-your-leptin/

About The Author

Mirsad writes all of his books in a unique style, constantly drawing connections between his past experiences and his reader's goals. This unique approach means that you can avoid undergoing the same injuries, frustrations, and setbacks that he himself has endured over the years. He can't produce the results for you, but what he can do is promise that you WILL reach your goals - guaranteed – providing you follow his tips and advice exactly as he outlines them in his books.

Made in the USA
Columbia, SC
13 March 2020

89131267R00063